Discovery Of A New World!

How Time Travel Really Works!

Book One

Edition 0.01

The calculation of optimized paths into the future for all of us.

Open questions from the bible, answered.

Michael von Khuon

Acknowledgment

A special

"THANK YOU!"

To ALL of YOU who helped
make this come true
and especially my family,
friends and of course
my wife Patrizia :-)

This would NEVER have been possible
WITHOUT YOU!

Table of Contents:

1. New definitions

When I was working at my master's thesis in philosophy at the University of Munich in Germany, my tutor asked me seriously, if I was inventing a new scientific language. That time back in 1990 I wondered, because to me everything seemed so clear, that everybody should understand. Today I see, he was right. A new world has to be defined by new terms, even if we had always already been living in it and only were used to different definitions of the terms.

Ignorance:
Remember just in case, if this gets too much: Ignorance does not protect against mistakes, punishment or even death! Take a break! Once you should know, but maybe not now!

Present: All beings have or had their own present!

Future and Past:
In this system of Time Travel you can find really a lot of future in the past! And past, present and future are relative. Your past can be somebody else´s future and vice versa.

Birth (rebirth):
We and our future are born every new moment in time again and again. This is about self-improvement for our own better future, how we can prepare the best possible way for our future. Rebirth should be understood here, that we are born already in a better future, if we made positive progress in just one of so many ways and don´t wake up in a worse situation of course!

Time Travel:

We all live in our own worlds and times, with our own present, past and future. Actually every word, every look and every exchange is traveling in time between different worlds and times. This might sound too easy, simple or trivial, but it turns out by far to not be the case, if only we consider the next important insight into this new world. This does not only hold for our living contemporaries, but also for our ancestors or any people of any time. Actually anybody, any named or not named being in any universe has its own past, present and future, its own history in its own world and time. The same holds for any book, any building, any star, any historic person, any animal, tree, ocean, friend, anything and anybody of any time. Now without doubt this system developing from the last ideas changes to real Time Travel in our own everyday world. This of course really means that we all have our own past, present and future and we all live in our own world and time. This especially holds for all beings of all times, even if they are alive OR NOT!

Death:

If we think about the future, death is quite a big subject there. And if we go for serious scientific investigations, we can´t omit it. Here the term "death" has always to be seen in connection with birth and rebirth. Every end means a new beginning. On the micro-level the "death" and "birth" of an instant is seen as a moment in time mostly changing to the worse or the better and never staying the same. Of course our investigations are first about our present changing to the better future, about fitness for our better future and about "passing the coming exams"!

It´s not now about going to heaven or hell in the end! It´s not about going to heaven or hell after Judgment Day! It´s about going to a better or a worse future NOW!

To put it easy: In the Bible the decision on the life in your responsibility is: heaven or hell. Looking at your life in the moment NOW, your responsible decision goes for a better or a worse future! Your life and your present are easily comparable from different perspectives. Your decision for the better result is important NOW!

2. Introduction

This E-Book matters! As a matter of fact it is important to make sure, that this E-Book addresses readers, who are ready for it!

If you bought this E-Book yourself or you consider yourself an adult, if you have reached your voting age or maybe you are a student at the university at an early age and your parents do allow, if you are a full member of your church or you are able and have to take full responsibility of your life, then you are alright to go ahead and to read and understand!

This E-Book is a test to check, if this world and time and You are ready for it. If You are not ready for it, You should be able to stop reading anytime at once!

But this E-Book is not only a test! It could serve as a basis for really a lot more, which already could be available, but still is waiting in the future! Nevertheless it now already reveals knowledge, which was unknown or possibly forgotten for thousands of years!

The subject is a kind of new, higher mathematics, described as simple as possible for the average Joe and Jane to tell them that they are Time Traveling already! By no means can it be complete as a system now, but just a test as described.

It gives certain hints that go far beyond anything that two famous German scientists, C. F. Gauss and Alexander von Humboldt, already knew in AD 1853, but nobody else has ever published more than that, because of the sheer difficulty of this subject.

No wonder! Nobody knew, until today that Gauss and Humboldt were investigating in Time Travel, even they didn´t know!

In this project we propose for all of us, to go for our best possible future! In a way it´s so great that it can´t be told here! You won´t believe! You can tell after reading!

Here you find a scientifically proven, mathematical system to calculate important dates in almost everyone´s future. Therefore you´ll be able to prepare better for your future and start optimizing your fitness for the future. This system tells you how Time Travel works and how to calculate and optimize your path into the future. This is of most vital interest for your very life and future! This is true and you should really know!

This actually is a new update on the history of science since AD 1854, which is 162 years now, not to forget the included new update on questions and answers from the Bible since Moses and John.

The first ideas of the system for the answers are presented here. OK, we know, there is a fine line between genius and insanity. And there we are now! But how complete can this system be to cover highest genius and deepest insanity. Both can be healed, if they come together and get normal again, but maybe on a new level. So, this is just an E-Book published here in 2016, but not just one like most of the others!

The content is about the known and the unknown and it intends to make the best out of both.

It's actually like: "Let's run it up the flagpole and see what happens." :-)

An opportunity for questions and answers will be given in the following forum, which already has many members:

http://www.futureok.net/forum/

The most important Q&A's will be considered in their own new section in the next edition of this E-Book.

3. How was this system discovered?

The first ideas dawn in your mind, when you realize that some terms we were used to understand differently, could certainly be understood in a new and by far better working way and system. This would deliver a lot of answers not known before until even today. This happens when you realize that a lot of terms are understood differently in different times.

Now there might occur the danger that all this might get too much at once for you!

In this case:

4. TAKE A BREAK!
**(To think about,
what is best to be done next!)**

Remember!

This is a short
E-Book,
covering decades
of investigations
about Time Travel,
that works!

To be able to take
an immediate break, to
be on guard and
flexible in your
decisions is a very

important ability in this new world of Time Travel, that you are about to discover!Just like in the discovery of any new world!

Some new definitions of "death", "birth", Time Travel, past, present, future, etc., that are used here have been explained from the view of the microcosm first:

Every moment the present is changing and becomes the past. But you'd better remember that every moment the future is changing to be the new present too.

This means that every moment is constantly "dying" to the past, while it is "newly born" from the future at the same time.

In short: "Everything flows" (old greek: πάντα ῥεῖ), but to and from different locations and directions in time and space! Now: This system is about actively going to a better future!

Your own future experience will have to prove, that in this new world of Time Travels, you will find a lot of certain dates in your very own future! With astronomical precision, you will find your own certain dates you never knew before and you should be prepared for in the best way you can. But how can you be prepared for dates that you don't even know about?

You will learn a lot, not only about your own future, but you will also gain the ability to prepare for those dates in your own future. With this knowledge, you will be able to improve yourself to better meet your future. You will start optimizing your fitness for the future, may be even in general!

By the way: A solution to "death", as the greatest problem in our future, will be provided here by the concept of "divide-and-conquer", that "is an algorithm design technique, that solves a problem by splitting it recursively into smaller problems until all of the remaining problems are trivial"[1], and then combines the subsolutions to get a solution to the original problem.

---

[1] An algorithm design technique applied to various algorithms, that solve a problem by splitting it into smaller problems until all of the remaining problems are trivial.
https://en.wiktionary.org/wiki/divide_and_conquer

5. Any initial hints to this system?

If you want to know something about the future and want to reach any goal, you ought to know that any time something could happen and you might definitely not make it! So you have to know something about that, what might hinder you from reaching your goal. Is it accidental? Is it fate? Can you change something for the better? We have to know, if our fate is guided by us, by someone else or a higher power! This way we might gain the ability to learn, what is the best we can do for our future.

The following story is so great!
We wondered already decades ago!

Read and listen yourself, think about it and get active! You might be able to imagine how we feel about it, if you think about the following:

"Is there an almighty God?"

And here this story begins!

Think about a 13-year-old pondering about dropping out of the protestant church, because he felt he was not taken seriously and then his whole family dropped out. His heavy fate made him think a lot more at age 23, about ten years later! His father had died at age 55, when he was twenty two, then his Great-Auntie a year later at 90 and he found himself alone, moved to some other city, so lost!

Still he wanted to make it himself, but he knew he had to find help and had to find a teacher he could accept.

He found one from another world, from the Himalayas and Trinidad and another from India and another, ..!

He learned and practiced meditation and Yoga in search of the sense of life and a possibly existing God!

He had to think seriously and he concluded: If EVERYTHING happened just by chance, there would be no final sense in ANYTHING, because EVERYTHING could easily be destroyed totally just by accident.

There really would be no sense in anything! There would be no sense in reaching any goal, because we might never reach it just by chance.

The path would be the goal!

But to him, it was not yet possible to believe or understand, what THAT really meant.

There must be sense in something, if not in everything, he thought, and in this way his search began.

Well, we don´t really know, he thought. But, if there is one God and we can make Him our friend or even realize that He might be our creator, the creator of all mankind since Adam and Eve, of all Jews, Christians and Muslims, this may be a fairy tale or our only chance to find a favorable path beyond this world and time, even beyond the reality of our life, unless we believe in another religion or in rebirth. Of course, deep in our mind, we know that there is something by far bigger than us, even if we forget it most of the time.

In this system presented here, we plan to be fit for the future, which certainly means being able to win against "death" finally, and then win a better life just the way it´s outlined in the New Testament in the Bible.

Don´t be afraid! "Death" AND "Rebirth" are defined in a new way here!

The first difference is that here we propose certain steps and skills, a new thinking, behavior and habits, to enable us to make positive progress in any way on the path into our optimized and best future.

In fact, winning against "death" means nothing else, other than to enable us to make our path into a better future, which in this way will be our rebirth from a worse past to a better future.

Of course we'll never be able to do this alone, but only with the appropriate help.

If you actually look closer, the past must die into the future. In this manner, our problem is by far smaller, than we thought before. Self improvement is about the "death" of the "worse" self and the "birth" of the "better" self. That 's more or less easy or difficult.

It depends on how developed your skills are in this field.

Specifically, it's a matter of preventing people making the same mistakes over and over again. It's about identifying mistakes and it's about making the best of our possibilities. Some people of course will think that this is as crazy as it can be, but as you easily may concede, to have a realistic chance to reach the best possible goal, you have to have in mind the "impossible", which might also be possible once in a while or just some time later. But here, fortunately it is the next step ahead :-) From the state of the art, there is most certainly only one way to make it for each and everybody! Well of course, as Christian preachers tell from the Bible, Jesus Christ was the first to make it and all Christians are called to take their cross and follow him.[2]

Actually the story that follows, is an update to the history of our world based on the Bible and more..! It is a story from the beginning of counting the years and days of our lives. The timeline covers the whole Bible from the Ten Commandments to the Book of Revelation, and goes ahead to

2 The Bibel. King James Version, Lukas 9:23-27

ourselves right where we are now, and even to our own most vital future.

From the Alpha to the Omega, the Bible tells us what to do and what not to do, what is right and what is wrong. And in the end, we will be judged about how well we did. This is a system that tells us what mistakes we should avoid and what's the best we can do.

And actually this new system we're going to introduce here, turns out to be a historically very well-founded system of optimized self improvement, derived from the Bible and the history of our world that will now be presented to the public for the first time.

This system can show the best way into the future for us and help us to preferably avoid the most pitfalls in our lives. It can calculate core answers and paths into our best future. It proves that we always have been traveling in time, however, probably in a sense we never thought about.

The first dimension of our system covers our reached age in different stages in relation and comparison to a certain age of really interesting people of our own history, of the history of our family, our country and the history of the world, counted in years and days.

It has to be admitted that this same kind of investigation has already been pursued by others, namely the famous German mathematician, astronomer, geodetics engineer and physicist Johann Carl Friedrich Gauss, who only revealed it in a private letter to his friend Alexander von Humboldt, Chancellor of the Order Pour le Mérite on December 7th, 1853. More on this soon!

It seems to us that since that time, no one ever was able to publish something ahead of these glimpses of great investigations of Gauss, as revealed in his letter mentioned above. Because of their old age of 76 and 84 in AD 1853, our fate did unfortunately not allow more to be published at that time, even until today. Only Prof. Dr. Karl Christian Bruhns published these letters on the occasion of the 100. anniversary of the birth of Gauss uncommented in AD 1877. Gauss himself by the way only survived this letter to Humboldt only by 443 days because of old age.

6. A system of Time Travel!

The start of this system was leaded originally from some different questions, and maybe Gauss investigated in a similar way, because his mother made it close to her 96th birthday already in 1839 just a few days before his own 62nd birthday. Our Forscher had also thought how his great auntie could make it to 90 years old, when his father only made it to 55 years old one year before her.

The first emerging questions our searcher here had a lot earlier at age twenty two:

1. How can I get ahead of my father in the same age comparison?

2. How can I celebrate my 90th birthday, like my great looking Great-Auntie?

These questions were not at all about Time Travel yet, but at least the first questions were present about calculating a path to a better future at that time.

The questions originated from a series of key experiences that explain quite something, e. g.: The 90th birthday of his Great-Auntie!

If you visit your Great-Auntie for her 90th birthday and are completely surprised at how really good-looking she is, you might easily find yourself wondering too: "Wow! If you look like that, you can make it to a hundred!"

However, she took a big breath, pressed her arms into her hips and said: "You first make it to ninety and then we talk again!"

Now he had to think a lot! Since he was close to his 23rd birthday and she was about four times his age, he remembered instantly, that his father had died the year before at 55! So he said nothing more and started thinking! Until he could celebrate his 90th birthday, really a lot could happen or come in between and he might not make it! If reincarnation worked, quite a few further lives might be needed to make it, he thought later.

Today, Time Travel-theory and practice is all logical and scientifically clear.

That time he and his Great-Auntie were 67 years apart, actually she was 67 years ahead of him, although together they celebrated her 90th birthday at the same time and place.

The following insights are developed from thinking about this incident: He concluded years later, that his Great-Auntie lived in her time and world and he in his own time and world.

She had her own past, present and future and he had his own. Both worlds and times were separate from each other more than 67 years.

To make this clear again: Obviously, they had both their own present, past and future, even if there were some common times of course. That is important in order to basically understand this new system of Time Travel.

The scientific summary tells us the following: We all live in our own worlds and times, with our own present, past and future. Actually every word, every look and every exchange is traveling in time between different worlds and times. This might sound too easy, simple or trivial, but it turns out by far to not be the case, if only we consider the next important insight into this new world. This does not only hold for our living contemporaries, but also for our ancestors or any people of any time. Actually anybody, any named or not named being in any universe has its own past, present and future, its own history in its own world and time. The same holds for any book, any building, any star, any historic person, any animal, tree, ocean, friend, anything and anybody of any time.

Now without doubt this system developing from the last ideas changes to real Time Travel in our own everyday world.

This of course really means, that we all have our own past, present and future and we all live in our own world and time. This especially holds for all beings of all times, even if they are alive OR NOT!

Thus, if You start dealing with dead people, the subject gets undoubtedly more difficult, even dangerous and even more, if you are not prepared at all.

Now of course we are reminded again of very important questions! Do you think now, that this world emerged only accidentally? Or could there be a creator or a universal intelligence?

If there is any remedy against "death", it is only God or maybe guardian angels, or any higher powers, energies or beings saving us and accepting us as worthy of their help. This tells us our own experience or the experience of others. This may well be even my own belief and experience and it´s following the same story, that is written in the holy books.

The chance of "death" winning against us is of course by far bigger than us winning the other way around only just by chance and without any other help. Who are we against "death"? This means: Alone we are lost! That´s why we need help!

What follows here is at least, that you should gain the capability first to immediately, anytime and anywhere, break off negative thinking and doing, and in this way, be able to instantly turn to positive thinking, talking or doing.

Learn what´s good and what´s bad for you! For example, first learn to meditate and to find positive support, if you think you are too weak for this following adventure.

There is no doubt you have to, if you once in a while you want to make it.

Or, what is vitally important to know: You reap what you sow and what you think, tell and do ist, even with your words, thoughts and deeds. Positive self control of our mind is obviously another desired skill, that is wanted here.

There is certain evidence, that this last advice is for advanced Time Travelers only!

The next advantage of this system is, that even the calculation of our future turns out not to be only a possibility but a reality in practice.

The same holds for everyone´s vital interest in changing their whole closer and distant future to the better.

To the contrary changes to a worse future happen most of the time only unconsciously and just by ignorance.

And here we get the tools to learn avoiding important mistakes we might soon be about to make.

We can even start calculating what we can do to go for our practically best future, because we know better what´s ahead.

To me there is no doubt that now there are answers found to Moses questioning the Lord in Psalm 90:12 from the English Revised Version: "So teach us to number our days that we may get us a heart of wisdom."[3]

3 http://bibeltext.com/psalms/90-12.htm

7. Any scientific background?

Our investigator´s studies of Computer Science with the minor subject Mathematics at the Technical University of Munich in Germany were overshadowed by his grief and his questions on the sense about the death of his father and then a year later, also his Great-Auntie.

The freedom of student life in Munich gave him absolutely every chance to find answers. The fact, that he had to find answers nobody had found or published before, became quite clear only much later in the course of his investigations. The deep grief which took possession of him was perhaps also a protection against so much truth that would have been too much for him too early.

Here a quote fits perfectly from Prof. J. Richard Gott[4]:

In the preface of his book, Time Travels in Einstein's universe, Prof. Gott writes that "people kept asking about the latest developments in the field of Time Travel and wanted to get information about it, because they were very serious about, e. g. whether it was possible to return into the past to save beloved people, who had died in tragic circumstances".

In his book Prof. Gott wrote that he took such calls very seriously. Partly he had written this book in order to answer questions like these. Another reason that Time Travel was so fascinating for him and his readers was,

---

4 Prof. J. Richard Gott, Princeton, Time Travels in Einstein's universe,
Houghton Mifflin Books 2002, pp. 9-10.

their strong desire for these most wanted answers!

This way of course anybody has the right to ask for the meaning of life and death and for a possible rebirth, especially after these beloved relatives or friends were lost from their own closest personal environment.

Our young researcher asked just the same questions, after his father´s and his Great-Auntie´s death, because they had been most important members of his closest family. And absolutely nobody around had any satisfying answers for him.

But real insights were still far away, even despite the fact, that later he was lucky enough to be really satisfied about the answers he found in the course of the years and decades of his research.

In the next important personal step he changed his main subject Computer Science, even his university and moved in the summer of 1982 to the faculty of Philosophy at the University of Munich in Germany and selected the minor subjects, Logic and Theory of Sciences and Statistics.

But still he followed his favorite studies outside the university to learn some interesting new visions of the world from India, China, Japan and the Himalayas.

At the university he was lucky enough that there was no limited study time yet, and he was thus at least for some five years able to study the meaning of life without temporal limit.

His search had become most important to him after the previous strokes of fate. In addition, in those years, almost all of his important new teachers came from the Himalayas and India to Munich, what developed as a lot of good luck on his path to the solution of his questions.

8. Is there an almighty God?

Again. If all this gets too much for you now, take a break! To be able to take an immediate break, i.e. to say "Stop!", is a very important ability in this new world of Time Travel! It can even save your life!

Because he had left the Protestant church at age 13, now after these hard strikes of fate, he wanted to find any first evidence about the existence of God. From his own point of view until the dawn of his most important questions, he had actually grown up without God.

His questions were fundamental to answer the question as to how he could survive until his own 90th birthday, because indeed, until then, everything possible could interfere and by any "accidental chance", he would not be able to celebrate his 90th birthday himself or even reach any new goal.

So gratefully he took the extremely favorable offer of the early 1980s at the University of Munich and made some very, very important experiences outside the university as a student of some yoga teachers and gurus from India, China, Tibet, etc..!

The decision as to whether life is governed solely to be accidental, if this world was only created by chance alone, was very easily made through his experiences from yoga and meditation.

Ultimately he decided that it was better to at least learn or experience anything about a real God. He wanted even to try to become a friend of God, according to the Qur'an or even a child of God, according to the Bible and the given Ten Commandments.

He later learned that these Commandments were made for a better future of all of us.

Indeed, while looking for a means to test the outcome of his actions, his emotional intelligence turned out to be a great tool to check, if he had done right or wrong. The random could hardly help him to the path to a better or the best possible life and future. In fact, he practiced meditation a lot, following the advice he learned since August 1981, according to his own demand, in order to ensure that he was on the right path to go.

The insights he got from meditation showed him in accordance with his knowledge and conscience, what very

probably was best and most important to be done next. This was the goal! He was on the path!

9. What made this thinking possible?

After he met and studied some important meditation teachers and their methods from 1981 to 1988, he found a yoga master who had been a member of the government of India. However, soon after that, the former Minister of Education and Science of Bavaria came back from government to the University of Munich and accepted the Chair of Christian world view, religious and cultural theory. This chair was right in the same house, one floor upward from where our protagonist studied his subjects of interest. And "accidentally" he sought for a professor to finish his Master of Philosophy at the University of Munich.

In the meantime, the University pressed students to finish their university degrees or to leave, because after a transition period, the unlimited time for study was then changed to be limited.

The story on how he contacted his future professor and major advisor is quite interesting in this context:

When he once wanted to find out about the program of the next semester on the black board of the seminar of his future professor, this professor joined him at the black board and also seemed very interested.

A short, lively conversation ended in an invitation for him to take a main seminar on the subject, "Past Future" as a test for a future cooperation. This topic pointed quite clearly to his later ideas on his new concept of Time Travel.

It was a major breakthrough, kind of his first conscious Time Travel, when he came across the family history of his own surname while researching in the library of the Bavarian state for his requirements for this seminar.

It was like his energy started flowing and getting hot, he started to perspire, and he saw his whole life passing by in seconds before his very eyes. He understood so much in seconds, especially why everything in his life had developed this way.

Involuntarily one of his first Time Travels had happened to him, amazingly including family history some 500 years ago. Now he was able to report to his professor that already in AD 1511 a member of his family had been appointed rector of the University of Ingolstadt in Bavaria and Professor of Ethics, and as well in AD 1523 Professor for Institutions. And the father of this member of his family was even more famous, because he had made history of justice as the creator of a book of law in the Holy Roman Empire!

This was exactly what was missing to start to finish his Master of Arts with the former minister of culture in Bavaria as his professor and major advisor.

Later he realized that here self-knowledge was in the true sense the first road to recovery. And actually this theory and practice of Time Travel as presented here delivers the same kind of self-knowledge for each and every one of us.

The subject of his master´s thesis was in 1990: "Terms and their developments as a source of historical knowledge!"

Of course the subject was not undemanding at all, but he had an encyclopedia of the history of terms at hand, which outlined and commented on the historical developments of important terms throughout the whole known western history.

However, his task for his thesis no longer seemed to be too difficult, because he was allowed to propose terms of his own interest himself. He had done a lot research on those chosen terms and had even experimented quite a lot on his subjects of interest.

But one day while he was working on his thesis, he noticed that his original question as to how he could celebrate his own 90th birthday, was not at all answered yet, even after more than ten years of study at the university.

With the subject of his thesis he had various histories of terms, which had gone through a number of developments, changed by important statesmen, philosophers and scientists in chronological order throughout the centuries.

Thus, for example, the earth had no longer been considered as the center of the universe since Kepler and Galileo, but slowly but surely was recognized as revolving around the sun.

What concerned his first, unsolved question, his minor subject of Logic and Theory of Sciences suggested that he at first should ask various philosophers with the help of their books, how he could celebrate his 90th birthday himself.

He really didn´t need to ask Descartes (*1596-1650, (who made it to 53 years, 19675 days)), Leibniz (*1646-1716, (70 years, 25703 days)), Kant (*1724-1804, (79 years, 29149 days)), Hegel (*1770-1831, (61 years, 22358 days)), because they did not manage to make it to their 90th birthday. (Sources on

Descartes, Hegel, Leibniz, Kant can all be found on Wikipedia, etc..!)

Descartes, Leibniz, Kant, and Hegel were ordered here chronologically after their birthdates, with respect to look at the developing history of terms and their impact in each interesting case.

This was not effective, if it was about the answers of his own guiding questions, which from his view were already far ahead of the questions concerning his master´s thesis.

But, if he wanted to find answers as to how he could reach age 90, the sequence of competence for older age would be different. It would be: Descartes (53), Hegel (61), Leibniz (70), Kant (79), according to their achieved age.

He was well aware that in this case of investigation all four philosophers came from different backgrounds, lived in different times and in different living conditions.

Descartes (53, *1596 in La Haye / Touraine, France died 1650 in Stockholm, Sweden), Hegel (61, *1770 born in Stuttgart died 1831 in Berlin of course in different circumstances), Leibniz (70, *1646 in Leipzig - 1716 in Hannover) and Kant (79, *1724 born in Königsberg, died 1804 in Königsberg).

It doesn't seem to be really useful to try to compare these four philosophers. But from his or anybody else's point of view with his question in mind, it is quite meaningful.

All roads lead to Rome and his road would be just one road with many steps, well-considered what's the best road and what's the best steps.

Early in the year 1990 he soon overlooked a future until and beyond the 90th birthday and sorted philosophers into the dimension of competence on their subjective property, which in his mind would be able to explain to him, how he could manage to get older and maybe reach his own 90th birthday.

Here a basic principle becomes clear which explains that all elders of all times were or are ahead of us, while they have or had reached an age which we did not reach yet. So in one way or the other, we might be able to learn from them, to make it to our own goal in the future.

None of these philosophers should be compromised, because we can hardly know their living conditions exactly like they could themselves, but in any case, Descartes could still have explained in 1650 how we might be able to make it to our 53rd birthday,

Hegel had accordingly in 1831 competence for 61 years, Leibniz in 1716 for 70 years and Kant in 1804 for more than 79 years of experienced life. (Sources on Descartes, Hegel, Leibniz, Kant can all be found e.g. on Wikipedia, etc..!)

Indeed, Hegel studied Kant and Leibniz because they were German philosophers earlier than him, but Hegel still did not reach his 62nd birthday after them.

So from the point of view of our system of Time Travels, Hegel´s competence in certain aspects did not reach theirs. Or maybe he was just more or less lucky?

We´ll know better ourselves, if we can make it to our own 62nd birthday.

Here, but not now, the concept of karma might be applicable and obviously should be discussed!

Don´t draw too many "noteworthy" conclusions from these correlations, because you don't know enough yet, in particular to answer the question: How could he celebrate his 90th birthday himself? This was, what he noticed while working on his master´s thesis in 1990.

In fact, all his previous official studies at university since 1979 had not specifically contributed much to answer this question. He had however, without realizing it, already collected a whole series of important hints, one after the other, for his most wanted answer!

Here by the way we should note that Palmer proposed in 1992: Common region: a new principle of perceptual grouping. [5] Therefore, the four

5 Palmer, S. (1992). Common region: a new principle of perceptual grouping. Cognitive Psychology, 24, 436-

philosophers mentioned above could be perceived as elements of a common region of philosophy, which extends over several centuries or millennia, but now supplies the given example, which is rather substantiated from logic, mathematical set theory and cognitive psychology.

Of course in the beginning of the investigation it was not adequate to find only a group of very few philosophers, which matched the prerequisites, to provide an answer to his own most important question.

There would have been only some, but by far not enough members in the group he was interested in.

So his subject of investigation changed right away from philosophy to all sciences, to enable him to find a lot more competent scientists to answer his question on how to make it to 90 years old. Again this very fast turned out to be another, but now incomplete approach.

Because of the incompleteness of his first approaches, he found immediately his next object of investigation: the whole history of mankind, which now seemed to provide enough examples, which would most certainly lead him to his wanted complete subject of investigation.

Now, with this almost complete source of all available scientists and non-scientists of all times, his possible advisers could be consulted through literature or by any other available means. And every time he arranged new "elements" into his groups he wanted to examine, according to the new law of the "common region" from the Gestalt psychology, even though this law was not published yet.

Now theoretically he had enough test persons in his list to find out how he could make it to his 90th birthday.

He had two persons in 1990 he knew personally: a lady born in 1898 from his yoga group, and who later made it to 98 years old, and a city hermit, born in 1894, who officially later made it to 110 years old, although there were rumours that he was much older.

However, his investigations had approached a turnaround, because he realized already in 1989 that he should not forget himself with all these researches.

In deed he found with himself the first signs of old age, despite he was only age 32. This was actually a very important turning point in his investigations!

10. Where are we all traveling in time?

Where did he then find himself in this new order of Time Travel? When even President George Bush Sr. had proclaimed a new world order in 1991, when German Unification and the end of the Cold War had happened and the eastern bloc fell!

Explanation of another "New World Order"!!!

In 1991 he was age 34 and he stood once again in front of the black board of the seminar of his professor. He wanted to see what was offered in the next semester. Almost the only subject there was actually the famous, German philosopher Hegel, in the seminar, the main seminar, the upper seminar, in the lecture, etc.

Of course this had to mean something! Thus, he asked himself where he would find Hegel in his list and where in relation to Hegel he would find his professor? He had built a sustainable list of all personalities known to him and classified them into the age each of them had reached.

Therefore, all future contemporaries would have to travel at the latest by Descartes (1650) in their 54th year, in their 62nd year by Hegel (1831), in their 71st year by Leibniz (1716), in their 80th year by Kant (1804), in their 85th year by Newton (1727), etc., etc (Sources on Descartes, Hegel, Leibniz, Kant, .. can all be found e. g. on Wikipedia, etc..!)

In this manner is the path through life from birth to the 100th birthday not at all linear but rather a zigzag course, which leads from aim to aim and in every case to new Time Travels. Besides, according to your own list, you might feel like newborn again and relieved after each passed critical date, because you have certainly passed this date forever! It simply depends on how comfortable you are to this new world of Time Travel and how we equipped you are with knowledge and experience to handle this properly. Besides noted, the term "forever" means of course that you now are consciously acting in eternity![6]

So actually numbering our days and the days of our neighbors in our system of Time Travel after Psalm 90:12[7] leads us to important knowledge about our and

6 *The Bible. King James Version, Luke 9:23-27*
7 The Bible, KJV, Psalm 90:12
"So teach us to number our days that we may get a heart of wisdom."

our "neighbors" future and enables us to prepare for it according to our basis of knowledge we have about it.

Especially this will help us to better understand even one of the greatest of the Ten Commandments of the Bible in the light of our working Time Travel: ´Love your neighbor as yourself.[8]

This Commandment holds for our system of Time Travels too, between all these worlds and times, and was never before seen in the light of Time Travel. Love is there, now between different worlds and times, and has always been Time Traveling too, just like intuitions, insights or discoveries or all our human perceptions.

But here travels LOVE truly from biblical times through time and ages, centuries and thousands of years TO US!

8 The Bible. King James Version, Mark 12:31

After his impressive meeting with his professor and major advisor our student found that Hegel had made it to 61 years and his professor was just sixty years old. This was amazing! He was stunned! This was an exact coincidence! He was alarmed!

In scientific terms this was a correlation, but it didn´t mean that it was a causal relation yet! Only if his professor acknowledged why he selected Hegel as main subject for his next semester, why he acknowledged Hegel as his future object of investigation in AD 1991.

This meant concerning his theory that his professor possibly had planned for Hegel and worked very intensely on his subject. And maybe he already knew the "new found system" of our investigator?

So of course he informed his professor of his amazing and so far-reaching discovery, because he had a lot of value on the response. His professor answered thoughtfully; for 10 seconds, 15 seconds he thought about it. Then he said: "If that is so, then you still have Mozart ahead."

His own reaction was the feeling that suddenly he had a lump, kind of a frog in his throat, as if he had a nasty toad to swallow.

Mozart may forgive him, if he is alive somewhere else, but Mozart did not make it to his 36th birthday and our researcher was age 34 and of course he wanted to make it to age 36 at least! Moreover, he had done research already for more than ten years on how he could be able to celebrate his own 90th birthday!

11. Earlier research approaches?

The above mentioned, noteworthy meeting reminds him of the letter of Carl Friedrich Gauss to Alexander von Humboldt from December 7th, 1853, which our investigator had discovered about sixteen years later on June 7th, 2009 on the internet. When he realized, what he found, t,his letter had our researcher kind of immediately "electrified", so strong that approximately the next ten minutes felt like half an hour. He could not and would not move! The feeling seemed like a most wanted and rarely felt before, extremely pleasant, positive current, like a really strong "waterfall" full of pure energy powering into and through his body and soul, which he really did not want to interrupt by no means and in not in any form.

He had found the scientific proof which he had searched so many years for, which in his mind had been there before, but had not been found yet.

Amazingly, Gauss had also kept lists about a slightly different subject, about the life expectancy of famous men (calculated in days). Thus Gauss wrote on December 7th, 1853 to his friend and chancellor of his order Pour le Mérite, Alexander von Humboldt:

"It is the day after tomorrow the day when you, my esteemed friend, go over into an area which still none of the coryphées of the exact sciences has entered, the day when you reach the same age in which Newton has closed his earthly career measured by 30766 days. And Newton's power was entirely exhausted in this stage: You stand there to the highest joy of the whole scientific world still in the full pleasure of your marvelous strength. May you remain in this pleasure many more years."[9]

This example indicates a constellation between Gauss, Newton and Humboldt, initially only regarding Newton´s and Humboldt´s lifetime counted in days by Gauss:

1. On Dec 7th, 1853 Carl Friedrich Gauss, *April 30th, 1777 Braunschweig - Feb 23rd, 1855 Göttingen, was in his 77th year (27979 days).

2. His friend Alexander von Humboldt, *Sep 14th, 1769 Berlin – May 6th, 1859 Berlin, was in his 85th year (30764 days) on Dec 7th, 1853.

9 Karl Christian Bruhns (Ed.): Letters between A. v. Humboldt and Gauss, Wilhelm Engelmann, Leipzig 1877. Letter No. 45 of Carl Friedrich Gauss to Alexander von Humboldt from December 7, 1853, page 67-68.

3. And Isaac Newton, *Dec 25th, 1642 / Jan 4th, 1643 jul./ greg. Woolthorpe-by-Colsterworth in Lincolnshire – March 20th, 1726 / March 31st, 1727 jul./ greg. in Kensington, actually made it to 84 years (30766 days) some 126 years earlier.

We can perhaps understand the enthusiasm of Gauss (*April 30th, 1777 - Feb 23rd, 1855), 77 years (28422 days), on Dec 7th, 1853, if we consider, what even Goethe (*Aug 28th, 1749 – March 22nd, 1832) at age 81 believed in his diary entry from June 24th, 1831 (WA III 13, 98) of Galileo Galilei (*1564 - 1642, 77 years (28442 days), and Newton, 84 years (30766 days), when he wrote:

"He (Galileo) died in the year when Newton was born. This is the

Christmas of our new time". (Goethe)[10]
(Sources on Gauss, Humboldt, Newton
can be found on Wikipedia!)
Now Gauss believed on December 7th,
1853 well to be able to celebrate that
Newton in two days would be outdated
by Alexander von Humboldt and that
this would be the beginning of again a
new time.
Indeed, Gauss didn´t formulate or
possibly didn´t know yet that the
appointment called by him for
Humboldt with Newton would concern
every person at the age of 30766 days!
Next question: Who would have the
good or bad luck to survive until the
age of 30766 days in a more or less

10 Goethes diary entry from June 24th, 1831 (WA III 13,
98)"He (Galileo) died in the year when Newton was
born. This is the Christmas of our new time". (Goethe);
WA III 13, 98. Tagebucheintrag 24. Juni 1831, Goethes
Werke. Weimarer Ausgabe (Sophienausgabe). 143
Bände, Weimar, 1887-1914. Abt. III: Tagebücher.

good or bad condition? Does all this really depend only on good or bad luck?

Of course not, I believe! And I know!

The proven fact now is that through this Time Travel principle standing out here, a whole new world of target dates for all people of all times can be calculated and predicted.

This did Gauss not mention in his letter and maybe he was or wasn't aware of it, but probably he was.

In any case, his letter was only later published by Prof. Dr. Karl Christian Bruhns in the correspondence between Gauss and Humboldt on the occasion of the 100th birthday of Gauss.[11] Gauss

11 Karl Christian Bruhns (Ed.): Briefe zwischen A. v. Humboldt und Gauss, Wilhelm Engelmann, Leipzig 1877. Brief Nr. 45 von Carl Friedrich Gauss an Alexander von Humboldt, December 7, 1853, page 67-68.

himself was known to publish only complete findings.

Important explanation: This is the first way rebirth works in Time Travel: After each "better or worse, but survived, critical date with a certain death," like Humboldt's with Newton's on December 9th, 1853, you feel more or less as if you are reborn again and therefore a new time and "life" begins for you!

You will actually be able to feel the difference of the energy-levels before your Time Travel date and after, if you make it. And it certainly has to do with fear before that date and gaining self-confidence after you made it!

Here we are reminded of: The Bible. King James Version, Job 28:28 "..

Behold, the fear of the Lord that is wisdom; .."[12]

This new found, crucial principle of investigation in this system of Time Travel means, that you learn to know, that the relationships between birth and death, day and night, black and white, light and darkness, sun and moon, a black hole and a white hole in the universe, and of course of yes and no, positive and negative, etc, for the sake of completeness of the whole, multipolar universe, always belong together as a whole single ONE. This way it is implied in the Chinese Yin-and-Yang-principle.

With this knowledge and common sense, you can always avoid mistakes better and be prepared for

[12] The Bible. King James Version, Job 28:28 "Behold, the fear of the Lord that is wisdom;"

future dates. You can make yourself fit for the known and unknown future.

The principle of the present is easy to describe by "being born" and at the same time "dying" in every single moment, which is completely self-evident and also nothing special, because we only rarely notice it this way.

From another view in meteorology again and again a high-pressure area follows after every low-pressure area and after every thunderstorm the sun shines again. Spring follows winter, summer follows spring, autumn and the next winter follow summer. Sunrise follows sunset, then the next sunrise, etc...!

If we experience those many small "deaths" just like small changes, like every moment "is born" and "dies" at the same time, so that we don't even notice, that the next moment is born already. We even don't grasp the meaning of the many small "rebirths", which are following those many small "deaths", so that the whole issue is not even really problematic any more.

This is the normal way of life and it's so smooth, that we even don't notice it, only maybe in meditation. In meditation we can even go beyond time.

With this wisdom in mind we see that life is a coming and going, with the special meaning and even the Commandment for us, to avoid errors and to do the best we can, from the choices to be made. Then the problem changes and becomes solvable, even if we can't take too much of it at once. Now, after the discovery of these Time Travels, a whole new world of dates for all people of all times can be calculated and predicted.

As outlined here, each and everybody is able using these means to better prepare for and optimize their future, avoid mistakes and go for a more desirable and of course better future, that is most certainly still unknown to us!

And if you don´t know how to make it to go through this system, because of lack of energy, there might well be another small book of great help: *Ancient Secrets of the Fountain of Youth by Peter Kelder.*[13]

13 Ancient Secrets of the Fountain of Youth by Peter Kelder.
http://lib.ru/URIKOVA/KELDER/Ancient_Secret_of_th e_Fountain_of_Youth-Peter_Kelder.pdf

12. Outlook

If you're still asking now: What is all this about? From the point of view of the believer, this is actually about an important part of the first books of the Bible and the Book of Revelation coming true.

Scientifically anything is only possible accidentally, if you don´t believe yourself nor follow the advice! So this is a call for positive action!

What is introduced here, turns out to be a historically well founded system of optimized self-improvement that is grounded on thousands of years of history of mankind and the Bible, Quran, Vedas, etc.!

Watch out for the next published products on http://www.futureok.net/ or by @timetrave on Twitter.

37 years of investigation cannot really be for free. You only get 100%, if You go 100% for it.

I can only recommend to your most vital interest that you check, what this is all about.

By the way: I consider this subject to be so important that I am working on it with the best possible accuracy. As time changes following updates will be needed, so that new versions can be published again at any time following the demand. It´s about the best possible future for all of us. Who would not be interested in their best possible future?

I am! That´s for sure! :-)

If you are not able to believe that much, you might best start going for the goals you can accomplish. That´s the way to improve your power of believing, which directly has an impact on your power of realizing something!

13. Literature

1. An algorithm design technique applied to various algorithms, that solve a problem by splitting it into smaller problems until all of the remaining problems are trivial.
https://en.wiktionary.org/wiki/divide_and_conquer

2. The Bibel. King James Version, Luke 9:23-27
http://bibeltext.com/kjv/luke/9.htm

3. http://bibeltext.com/psalms/90-12.htm

4. J Richard Gott, *Time Travel in Einstein's Universe*, 2002, Houghton Mifflin Books, pp. 9-10.

5. Palmer, S. (1992). *Common region: a new principle of perceptual grouping.* Cognitive Psychology, 24, 436-447.
http://www.ncbi.nlm.nih.gov/pubmed/1516361

6. *The Bible. King James Version, Luke 9:23-27* http://bibeltext.com/kjv/luke/9.htm

7. *The Bible. King James Version, Psalm 90:12 "So teach us to number our days that we may get a heart of wisdom."* http://bibeltext.com/psalms/90-12.htm

8. *The Bible. King James Version, Mark 12:31 'Thou shalt love thy neighbour as thyself.`* http://bibeltext.com/mark/12-31.htm

9. Karl Christian Bruhns (Ed.): *Briefe zwischen A. v. Humboldt and Gauss,* Wilhelm Engelmann, Leipzig 1877. Brief Nr. 45 von Carl Friedrich Gauss an Alexander von Humboldt, December 7, 1853, page 67-68.

10. Goethes diary entry from June 24th, 1831 (WA III 13, 98) "He (Galileo) died in the year when Newton was born. This is the Christmas of our new time". (Goethe); WA III 13, *98. Tagebucheintrag 24. Juni 1831,*

Goethes Werke. Weimarer Ausgabe (Sophienausgabe). 143 Bände, Weimar, 1887-1914. Abt. III: Tagebücher.

11. Karl Christian Bruhns (Ed.): *Briefe zwischen A. v. Humboldt and Gauss,* Wilhelm Engelmann, Leipzig 1877. Brief Nr. 45 von Carl Friedrich Gauss an Alexander von Humboldt, December 7, 1853, page 67-68.

12. *The Bible. King James Version, Job 28:28* "And unto man he said, Behold, the fear of the Lord, that is wisdom; and to depart from evil is understanding."http://bibeltext.com/job/28-28.htm

13. *Ancient Secrets of the Fountain of Youth by Peter Kelder,* 1939, 1985, 1998, in the Internet or http://lib.ru/URIKOVA/KELDER/Ancient_Secret_of_the_Fountain_of_Youth-Peter_Kelder.pdf

14. Legal information

This copy is a copyright property from and by Michael von Khuon, whose unauthorized spreading, also in extracts, is observed, persecuted and traced under criminal, civil and any other applicable law.

Epub ISBN 9784409525074 Version 0.01

Author: Michael von Khuon
82041 Oberhaching / Germany
EMail: discovery@futureok.net
Internet: http://www.futureok.net/
My blog: http://www.futureok.net/blog/
My forum: http://www.futureok.net/forum/

Don´t forget: There are several opportunities mentioned above, where you can get news from this source!

Despite of careful check the author can assume no liability about the information provided in this copy. The examination of the single information is incumbent upon every single reader. He holds a master degree of arts in philosophy, logic, theory of sciences and statistics from the University of Munich / Germany since 1992. He is a web designer since 1998. He had been investigating on this subject for 37 years. Since AD 1877 and even since Moses in the Bible nobody published anything on this most difficult subject before!

Munich / Germany, September 14th, 2016, 5:25 p.m.